T0162364

HEADY BLOOM

Andrew Faulkner

COACH HOUSE BOOKS, TORONTO

first edition

 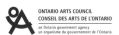

Published with the generous assistance of the Canada Council for the Arts and the Ontario Arts Council. Coach House Books also acknowledges the support of the Government of Canada through the Canada Book Fund and the Government of Ontario through the Ontario Book Publishing Tax Credit.

LIBRARY AND ARCHIVES CANADA CATALOGUING IN PUBLICATION

Title: Heady bloom / Andrew Faulkner.
Names: Faulkner, Andrew, author.
Identifiers: Canadiana (print) 20210298308 | Canadiana (ebook) 20210298332 | ISBN 9781552454435 (softcover) | ISBN 9781770567160 (EPUB) | ISBN 9781770567177 (PDF)
Subjects: LCGFT: Poetry.
Classification: LCC PS8611.A85 H43 2022 | DDC C811/.6—dc23

Heady Bloom is available as an ebook: ISBN 978 1 77056 716 0 (EPUB), ISBN 978 1 77056 717 7 (PDF)

Purchase of the print version of this book entitles you to a free digital copy. To claim your ebook of this title, please email sales@chbooks.com with proof of purchase. (Coach House Books reserves the right to terminate the free digital download offer at any time.)

for Bob Faulkner
and Martha Nash

TABLE OF CONTENTS

ON VISIONS

Awareness
bunched in the middle.
A low whine

as when a propeller
slices a layer of air.

Hildegard saw it before
she knew what it was.

Migraine sufferers report
a variety of sensations
that range in intensity

and duration. Dense
in the middle and hazy

at the edges. Julian of Norwich
had visions of love, which many

good people know not to exist.

Veronica Giuliani admitted
the heart is weak
and made hers a holy

steel vault. Narrow the eyes just so
and sight goes all wrong

and everywhere. When a tooth
is bad you can fill it

or pull it, those are the options.
But first you've got to know

what you're working with.
Catherine of Bologna catalogued
the soul's fangs and claws.

Veronica Garcia and Marci
Guinto and Josyp Terelya

and Branca Cepo and Veronique Demers
and especially dear Dory Tan

witnessed Our Lady in a field
in Marmora, Ontario, though maybe
what they saw was faith bunched

tight, a clump in the brain.
As when desire

manifests as lie. You've got
to cut through the bullshit,

is the gist of it. Starving oneself
produces both notable
and subtle effects.

Close your eyes and archangels
descend upon noun and verb.

Teresa of Ávila saw herself
shut in a closet, which is

a metaphor but seemed to her
a literal hell. Stay in one place
long enough and the absence

of change may cause a blip
in perception. To be so close with one's

mind that you're bound in it.
When blood comes up

it's a sign of something or nothing.
The heart knows which

and is often wrong.
Lidwina said an impoverished spirit
gleams like incandescent metal.

Some days it's kiss me
with blood and effluvium

and a weather of general feeling.
As good and true a sensation

as any. All sorts of things
can happen in the frontal lobes.

An aura, a hazy sense of purpose.
Birds blacken and fall from the sky.

Cardinal symptoms stand like vandals
at the gate. Though nobody's

really there, are they?
It's the uncertainty that gets you.

In accordance with a dream,
Sigfrid dragged three severed heads

across the mission field.
To have one's work squeezed

in a vice. Sigfrid saw an angel
as sure as you're reading
this. We know what we know,

though reconstruction is a problem.
Premonitory symptoms could be nothing.

Probably are. And yet.
Faust saw the devil

and Faust is made up.
Not to say the devil's not real.
Abstraction accumulates

in the body until made definite.
A fever dream, a bit of coke

in the night's false bottom.
A faint droning unfolds

behind the eyes and an unpleasant
sensation wriggles free.

Throw salt over your shoulder
because it could be worse.
A migraine is a locked box,

smoke against a wall.
When vision goes black,

that's when you worry.
Raymon Llull saw Christ

pinned in the air. What should one
do with the information

one receives? Juan Diego was told
to gather flowers, so he gathered flowers.

Light and sound beget a need
beyond reason. From there,

how well can you read a map?
When someone offers a competing

vision of life, listen up.
Long periods of silence could be a matter

of light and density. A brain clot.
Senses frayed, the air full of ghosts.

Anne Catherine Emmerich
saw the Holy Trinity as concentric
circles. A wheel within a wheel.

The pain begins at the centre
and extends in all known directions.

Anne followed the rules
and suffered much. Poet Clemens

Brentano circulated a rumour
Anne's a bride of Christ. But poets
make stuff up. Figurative rain

on a literal grave. The sensation
could be a headache only.

To obsess is a mistake.
What's not to believe? Suffering

and ascendance require the same work.
The literature is clear: these things
happen all the time.

One is advised not to argue
with the extraordinary persistence of vision.

Bridget witnessed light rearranged,
as if presence were a matter

of illumination. Consider the onset.
The extraneous symptoms.
Andrea dei Conti was much troubled

by demons. Aren't we all?
Conti's visions were routine,

common as a crow's dark throat.
You get used to anything.

Villana de' Botti spied a demon
in the mirror where her face

should've been. Something's there
or it isn't. A fact of shape,

orientation, location.
You see what you see.

The head thickens, sight is swept
clean of being. John Donne understood
his demise as a maid knows

the end-state of a room they're cleaning.
A bedsheet, a number burning

brightly. Grey slate and sunshine.
All of this in a literal sense.

A feeling floats free of context
in a way one might call 'fucked up.'
Maria Bolognesi was puppeted

by the devil and begged the saints
to free her. These things don't just happen.

Pelagia of Tarsus was burned to death
and the Benedictines say she didn't

even exist. You see the problem with belief.

Anyone can suppose they've heard
dogs barking, telephones ringing,
a name being called.

Mary whispered the future in Helen Aiello's ear.
In a crowd of sounds, you pick up on things.

Attention slips amid brain regions.
Metaphysical cloth is balled up. A lesion

exerts itself. Crystallized light tossed
like dice across a great white sheet.

Gemma Galgani staved off the devil
and received a message

from You-Know-Who. She was punctured
by a brain tumour or a crown of thorns,

does it matter which? She felt it
all the time, you understand.
The pathology, if that's

what it is, proceeds
like going down two steps

at a time. Space gets tight, it feels like.
Francisco and Jacinta saw the Virgin

Mary and died thereafter.
Shape and pattern form a latticework,

the density of which is subject to change.
Desire relocates to another quadrant.
From there it's anyone's guess.

The head bends liberty to its mean,
mean will. Peter appeared to Agatha

in prison and mopped up her blood.
You break a glass,

you get a broom.
Eustace saw a crucifix lodged

in a deer's forehead. Just like that.
Ditto for Hubertus. You have to go

forward under incredible circumstances,
let the mind's needle and thread

stitch everything up.
You see how one gets lost in it.
A sense of someone looking over

your shoulder. A sheet of ice
shattered by the hull of a ship

whose flag is unknown.
A brittle crackle

signifies a desperate
idea climbing out,

a migraine advancing in a mob of light.
Catherine Mattei saw holes in her hands.

Catherine Labouré saw the beating heart
of Vincent buoyed above her.

Catherine of Genoa was buffeted
by God's love. It doesn't end, does it?
The world trembles in the mind's eye.

And the mind, as you know,
suffers a certain degree of deception.

Being is shaken, disordered.
And if you stay with the shakiness

through its conjugations? Who knows.
Joy is episodic. Comes from anywhere.

Dostoyevsky testified to a happiness
unthinkable in a normal state.
Though anything carried

to its logical extreme becomes
depressing. Joan of Arc wept

when her visions left. Beauty's like that.

In certain conditions it can't be seen.
Like light. Like nothing at all.

Padre Pio believed the love of God
is inseparable from suffering,

which is a reasonable response
to suffering. To progress in severity,

as when the saints march
through a hole in the sky.

Some days the Lord's name
is a weather vane. Some days

it's the river you drown in.
Reports say vision goes cloudy,

the world diffracts,

then comes together
in a great band of light.

THE CASE FOR ADVIL PRESENTS ITSELF

First headache shows up like whoa.
Whistles through switch grass,

sedge, wheat-like prairie
June grass, a spread of bottlebrush

and my mind's declensions of thin pine.
What flesh extends from.

My head hurts. Is it swollen?
I think it maybe is. And what's

this rough seam, these roses and filament,
over which I can run my thought's thumb?

This is all just interior talk, mind you,
rumour of layoffs, downsizing,

exploring the future at length.
That from which flesh extends.

My head considers its freestone pit.
A condition's no good unless it persists.

LONG HAUL

Driving for a week now and always
the tires' reedy come-on-out voice.
You're in it for the long haul,

through elastic sunlight and motels
that approach well-made beds
per their provincial ideals.

Heart's never quite in your possession
when you wake. Resting in the next room, maybe,
is what it's like. Takes a few minutes to find it.

In Arkansas, a motor lodge resolves in watery
dark, in a sweep of fingerpaint children use
to indicate something certain in their mind.

Even the idea of driving at that point. The air
shocked with rain. The air descending like a statement
of fact. The view broken up by more view.

TERMS OF SERVICE

We begin as we are.
Let us sketch the contours
of a relationship, mutually agreed
upon if not drafted in unison.
To concur, in situ, on common terms.
Everything is fine. Revisions are possible.
Let the lawyers practise
their craft. We are creatures of love
and ambition and there is no future
state that cannot be resolved
in the future. You know what
everything is. Give us the goods
as we too give you the goods.
The terms of service reflect
light in all directions. Fine,
everything, all of it. The terms
are geological, the services thermic.
Thin wires in a smoke alarm.
There is a box to be clicked and why not.
Agree and everything is fine.

PARANOID ANDROID

Wakes up in winter. What time is it?
Set in ice, looking up at the bottom

of the world. The clock
tracks eternity. Thom, who is

the tinkle of glass on pavement,
hears water whisper.

He's sure of it. But when it's quiet
like this, like the open mouth of a vase,

he feels the air work him over.

In whose heart a fact hides
even from itself.

Open a door and there's the night,
slinking around like a bass line's
gravel-throated slander.

Thom is a gated vista. A financial district.
The last Blockbuster. An imperative

on all frequencies: renounce what you know.

Renounce what you know.

A cipher, a hinge, brushed steel.
Thom's attention is a white boat.
It's taking on water.

What would it mean to think straight?
Thom wants to know.

First rain. Then snow.
Every day feels parachuted in.

Dear Thom, who insists like a piston.

A thought slips from formation,
decamps to a new country

whose anthem is silence.

The signs Thom's born under. Events happen.
Freedom is a problem you wouldn't believe.

An engine turns to no accord
and turns

and keeps turning.
Little yarn-ball of noise.
Builds a hall of sound.
The stars crack their knuckles

and say, 'Pay your rent and you'll be fine.'
Say, 'Touch my sister and I'll kill you.'

After snow, rain again.
Then something indeterminate.
Imprecise.

Here in the crackle of glass
stitching back together.
The world belongs to those

who help themselves.
Thom wants to help.
When Thom presses his ear to a wall

he can hear Thom on the other side,
listening in.

A great electric wall of cocaine
and good times, nothing,
nothing wrong here.

Like kissing an angel.
A Xerox, a dizzy spell,
a pearl. In a forest of nostalgia

the nineties claw and wail.
Thom wants to get better
but doesn't know how.

PRECAUTIONARY MRI

A back-country flyover looking for exactly what?
It's embarrassing to worry in detail

but here I am imagining all bad things.
A light breeze passes through the body

like a wink at the devil.
Picture the devil winking back

and there will be no surprises.
When there's a knock at the door

I'll know who's there.

WHAT ADVIL GETS UP TO

Advil rolls up its sleeves:
'We gonna get started or what?'

From spit and straw, Advil assembles
amphetamine's scarecrow cousin.

Advil sucks its teeth as it thinks.

Advil is thick,
as always Advil is thick,
with representation.

Advil, coated in gypsum dust,
asks: 'What's an empty room
supposed to look like?'

In a Moleskine, Advil notes
the capacity for feeling hasn't changed
but the field of sensation narrows.

Advil makes a jerkoff motion as I sleep.

Advil shows a Polaroid of me
to the news camera: 'It's gruesome
that someone so handsome should disappear.'

Advil is always in the process
of rolling its sleeves.

Three days on Wikipedia 'fiddling with dates.'
Advil swears it's just documenting facts, sir.

At the early hours' threshold, Advil
asks: 'Why not you?'

This is what it's like, if you can believe it.

At the corporate retreat, Advil insists
on the profound, the meaningful.

But why not me? Advil tickles
my thigh: 'Want to interrogate the present?'

Advil's clean lines are appealing, but no.

LICHTENBERG CINEMA

The dark collects our empties, empties you of preference.
Did you mean 'What is the condition of a problem
if you are the problem?' in a good way?

Up in the fragrant rafters, a bunch
of uncanniness emerges. Could this go on forever?

Along the order of magnitudes, a glyph, tape loops.
As in the difficult dream the dark touches us up.

Please feel free to cue or cut the figure-ground relationship.
Sheet lightning and large-dropped summer rain in short forays.

You set out from consciousness – Damn. I've lost it.
Earlier you asked if I would enter the data like a room, well,

it seems that your data does that. A brain left lace
from age or lightning. Your lack of whatever.
At 20 hertz it becomes touch. This could go on forever.

GERIATRIC MILLENNIAL VIBES ON NOSTALGIA

Listen: I got the flavour for the fever.
Listen: I'd like to be someone
    who believes the past resides
               in a reachable place.
So I track an idea by its direction.
To be funky as a bomb over Baghdad
    or a missile over Kosovo.
Wisp of cloud in the shape of a dollar sign,
a shadow over
       a pornography of snow.
Recall that 'Informer' was played everywhere
and a semi-charmed decade hinged
on the relationship between money,
               which is a problem,
and problems, which bob in the eddies
of compound interest.
     Ah, the good times: those were
the good times. So listen: Can I kick it?
    My toddler wants to know,
repeats it, endlessly, can I kick it can I kick it can
I kick it, both question and answer,
       signal of a signal,
to be given a sign
     and then hit by it, again,
   again, baby,
one more time.

DUPLICATE WORLDS

The headache divides the patient
in half. Now the patient is in two
places at once.

Please, the patient would like
to be resewn. By whose hand,
whose needle? The patient isn't picky.

The patient is a buoy whose prayer
is a tide. Can the buoy drown?
The patient expects to find out.

Is Advil also a patient?
The patient has not considered this.
Advil has symptoms. A morphology,

a path of progression.
It can worsen.
What happens to the body

when it crowds itself out?
The patient is purple
with wondering, shadow

of a shadow's edge.
Disease is a condition
that afflicts the living.

The patient would like to keep living.
How to be a symptom of living,
the patient would like to know.

A FEVER DREAM MAY ARRIVE DESPITE THE ABSENCE OF A FEVER

with several lines from These Possible Lives *by Fleur Jaeggy,*
trans. Minna Zallman Proctor

So what if *Thomas De Quincey became a visionary*
in 1791 when he was six years old? My spirit

walks at night among the ditch lilies and litter.
I too am heard *emerging from the ominous*

murk of dreams. Despair is riotous
in the right body. Keats was *seized*

by the spirit of the time
and love may wield a knife

too close to the face.
Let me tell you the shapes

a spirit may take. A number, aflame,
travels a great distance,

from glinting crags
to the holy here-and-there.

A fever may act as a tuning fork,
or as a hastily chalked pentagram.

Such are the body's ways and means.
Marcel Schwob *suffered from a brain fever;*

the mind swings dreams like a censer.
Smoke may signal the onset of fire

or its end. When the spirit takes
no shape at all: that's when you worry.

ADVIL DRIVES AROUND THE BLOCK

I know Advil by the pitch and sweep
of its headlights, false daylight in the dead dark.
A pair of halogens conspire to make an object visible.
Tracks across a field of presence and absence,

trace of light beyond the usual range.
We measure ghosts by their ghostliness.
And Advil, which haunts my simple door?
The difference between real and manufactured

origins. Focus, when the mind wanders.
The brain runs on twenty watts of electricity
and greets you according to custom.
A boy in Saudi Arabia is jailed for blogging

and my breath fogs the car's what-do-you-call-it.
Advil's dark sedan cruises this block and the next
as each porchlight executes its function.
Leather seat can't help but creak. What's it saying?

ON BABIES

A baby born at twenty-four
weeks may weigh just over

a pound. At twenty-five weeks,
tubes and sanitation protocols.

A crook of gears. A specialist places
their trained hand on a shoulder

to indicate such are the odds.
At twenty-six weeks a baby continues

to extend in known directions.
As likely to live as any slash of hope.

At twenty-seven weeks a baby is a tiger,
tiger burned all through. Tangle

of jungle mind. A surfeit of conditions
under close observation. Attributes plotted

on a spectrum. At twenty-eight
weeks – look, twenty-eight weeks

isn't bad. Face almost recognizable,
could be yours. Twenty-nine

weeks, yes, thirty weeks, yes.
A week goes by and the baby's not here,

it's enough to make you cry in reverse.
Still, the thresholds of necessary

and sufficient are unclear.
As plagues begin with rats and fleas

and sermons emerge from a head
of metaphysics, so is a baby born.

A window blind undrawn.
A postcard from another

continent: wish you were
here and good fucking luck.

SELF-PORTRAIT FROM ANOTHER ROOM

Two arms, two legs
and arranged,
like most appliances,

along a central axis.
A thicket of teeth and blood
for the taking. A real angel.

A real retractable-cord type.
If a clay vessel's useful
because it's hollow, what's it

to him that he's full
to the brim? He thinks
his thoughts as one

scoops ice cream.
Poor sweet porthole
soul. Poor jar of piss

longing to be vinegar.
Two eyes in his face
and face square

in his head.
Always next door
to where he is.

ON BEING

Exactly as advertised. Centre-matter stuff.
Heart of the mind's eye without heart

or mind or eye. The subway's
a cistern of it; jostle of arrival

and departure, great glut of strangers
gathered and hauled away...

but I'm being dramatic,
gambling with the facts at hand:

who among us hasn't turned ashen
when the cab they've flagged travels

at a despairingly slack pace. You want time
but you get place. You know what I mean

but can't point to where the knowing
goes. That's what being's like.

IPO

The IPO is a body of light,
the brochure says, crisp

as a Bud Light and steady as she goes.
The IPO asks me to think of a thesis

that renders itself obsolete. The IPO
asks about a future that claws

its hours back, would I like that?

Would I like a metaphor to diffuse
some obvious and fucked-up tension?

I would, right? The IPO is like
'C'mon, man' and points to the horizon.

It asks me not to split my attention
but I know not how.

I have nothing for the IPO.

I am sorry.

The IPO is sorry.
Hordes of faces, in sleeplessness,

all sorry.
The evening apologizes

in a profuse bloom. It's obscene,
how sorry it is.

ADVIL HAS BIG SUMMER PLANS

At Tim Hortons Summer Camp for Kids with Pain,
the dark is inflamed. On a good night

the headache leaves its bunk
to pace the obviously staged moonlight.

Pressure convenes in the brain's general vicinity.
Peach that won't ripen, then turns, worsens.

With an oversized watch and chemo eyes
the headache returns to bum a light.

'Let's go,' it mouths – but where?
On a bad night this goes on for years.

Here Advil breaks the fourth wall, waves
a paintbrush, admonishing, 'Less Goya, more Bruegel.'

Advil lights a sparkler and outlines its promises
in the air: an unencumbered hour,

a fix for the hitch in an essential gear.
When you live in a Hank Williams song,

invite the big dogs to displace
the small dogs. Things get swell

and sweller. Dear liquid-gel,
you'll fit right in.

ON HOT DOGS

An ash-voiced blurber says a new book
is heart-wrenchingly rendered.

Its components are bent
to the mean of taste,

like a hot dog, reproduced
ad nauseam and groomed

by need's coarsest comb.
Arrives by the truckload,

shadow in hunger's daylight.
Tastes so real you'll swear
it was once alive.

REC CENTRE GYM

Where citizens exercise the right to produce sweat.
Subject and object of class theory meet

in adrenaline's high fever, among set
and repetition. An altered ratio of mass

and fat – they want it. Night-shifters,
the working poor, office folk

with modest pensions. The big-boned.
The people of FM soft-rock-land who labour

under good health's auspices. Autodidacts
and the shy consulting charts and diagrams

on how to lift oneself into ideation.
Elliptical enthusiasts who love the high-point

view of the pool, briny with chlorine.
Musclework and pain like fire at the door,

hygienic spray, a drop-in rate,
why are you doing this? Admit the future

will never arrive.

DOLLAR SHAVE CLUB

Summer and the heat is unbearable,
my face unbearable, the cost of dragging

metal over my skin unbearable.
If there's a good deal, Occam says

we should take it.
In the face of competing principles

we should shave with the grain.
I cannot access beauty

but I can save a dollar,
and an honest life

in the black is no mean thing.
I resolve to cut evil at the root.

To know a good deal when I see it.

ADVIL CLUMSILY RETELLS NORM MACDONALD'S MOTH JOKE FROM *THE TONIGHT SHOW WITH CONAN O'BRIEN*

'A moth walks into a podiatrist's office,'
Advil begins as it yanks the rip cord

on an impression of Norm Macdonald
that labours like a train hauling coal

through a minor landscape,
the clenched teeth, the grinding

mental effort to dig up
a joke so perfect

it eats you whole.
The foot doctor asks,

'What's the problem?'
 Here's the problem:

The moth's in a funk.
'I walk here and there,'

Advil says in the moth's voice.
The moth's wife is a flicker

of her former self.
The moth's daughter caught cold,

died, life is fragile.
And the moth's son,

oof, is the living reflection
of Dad's despair.

The poor podiatrist,
he's just listening

as Advil explains things
are, in a word, 'not good.'

Advil takes a moment
to note the YouTube video

of Norm Macdonald
on *Conan* is classified

Pets & Animals; some pills
are easier to swallow than others.

But the joke.

The son, daughter, wife,
malaise, it's enough to drive

a lepidopteran to the brink.
Naturally, the moth owns a firearm,

gun's on the nightstand,
and one can hear the bullet

pacing its chamber as the moth
works out his dilemma:

how to go on living
when living feels like death.

Advil pauses to acknowledge
this bit's success is predicated

on a mutual recognition
of how well and truly fucked

we are. 'In a cosmic sense,'
Advil says, 'we're all the moth.'

But the joke.

It's dead. Advil's wielded
explication like an ice axe

and the joke's gone
the way of Trotsky,

theory murdered by praxis,
and what's left is the moth,

who's staring down
a barrel-shaped dread,

and you, dear receiving end,
who must hold this shaggy

moment and hack through
the fact that Advil's lost the plot,

can't stick the punchline,
as the podiatrist has no clue

how to shoo the moth
from his office.

Some jokes are so clear
they aren't really there.

And then Advil,
Norm, the podiatrist,

they know what to do,
they've got it,

a light goes off.

THE ATRIUM

Of course I know the song, the handshake,
the shorthand, the definitive emotion
of our time, the key and register
and right sequence of notes. Yes
I know the dress code, the active
ingredient, the place on the corner,
shadows that drain like spinal fluid
when headlights flick on.
I know barns where water pools in moonlight.
Bills that accumulate like rumours.
The Subway sandwich artist
who slackly polices the soda dispenser.
I know when the atrium is empty, the newspaper
stand unmanned. I know which YouTube videos
to disown and which to gather like glitter.
The correct compounds in forgetting,
the metronomic click across a burnished
floor. I know a lobby is a cavern of exits.

SCROOGEMCDUCKSWIMMINGINGOLDCOINS.GIF

Money. A blue wireframe. Hazy lighting.
Greetings from flat-bottom leisure days.

    To be a veil, an object must obscure
    an object behind it.

      'If love be rough with you, be rough
      with love,' but for money.

        The censer-like dream: an arch,
        a glass tower at dawn, an idle car.

Money again. A Venn diagram:
what's governed by law, by a higher law.

    Preposition, noun, strained through abstraction.
    To approach each breath as a question.

      Scrooge at the gate with sparkles,
      spigot in the eyes of the Lord.

Literal rain on a figurative grave.
Buy anything and poof, it's yours.

Money again. Arrives like the cool
side of a pillow and leaves like the same.

To divest of specifics. To circulate
the silhouette of a knotty concept.

A bathing suit, a theory of water,
the angel of history, but for money.

In a body of currency, the deeper
you go, the deeper you are.

Money again. Photo-shoot style,
light and more light. Light by the kilo.

To haul value from one moment to another.
Problems have a freedom you wouldn't believe.

Emerging, mid-loop, as a signal of a signal.
Two fingers and a thumb make a circle when they rub.

A threshold of paper. Double-blind metaphor.
A veil is anything that gets in the way.

GUNS N' ROSES PINBALL MACHINE

The bus hums in a low register
and will not open its doors. The driver

attends to his dashboard and refuses
eye contact. This is – Kelowna?

Merritt? – where the promises pile up.
A vending machine sells sugar and carbs

to the malcontent, the en route.
The overcaffeinated shadow a pinball

machine with an upright display featuring Axl
airbrushed into a half-decent state.

Its audio is proximate and the gutter
will slay you. The game darkens the depot

like a sweetly blackened eye.
Skin discolours where blood convenes.

It's not quite pleasing. But whither the fun
in a jungle of leaving.

ADVIL FOLLOWS STAGE DIRECTIONS BRIGHTLY

ADVIL: [frontier town at dusk]
ME: [hooves on the road]

M: [gunshot]
A: [cash register bell]

A: [pillow fort]
M: [pillbox]

M: [cardinals at the gate]
A: [an oral history of hinges]

M: [tinsel]
A: [cellophane]

A: [the seven stages of success]
M: [the definitive emotion of our time]

M: [blood on the temple]
A: [blood on the sheets]

A: [keys shaken at the dark]
M: [face like a lock]

A: [refresh]
M: [like]

A: [getting lit]
M: [lighter by the second]

A:
M: [refresh]

AMERICAN SONNET FOR MY PAST AND FUTURE ARIEL

This one goes out to daddy. In the picture
I have of you, you are the color of a sucker
punch. I am sick of baggage. On some level,
I'm always full of Girl Scout cookies, marble-heavy,
a bag full of God. My skin bright as a remix
of 'Pony' by Ginuwine. I turn and burn.
So this is what it means to have love
set you going like a fat gold watch.

My hunch is that Sylvia Plath
was not especially fun, a buddha,
all wants, desire falling from me
like a shootout in an African American
Folk Museum. I am a lantern. I was raised
by a beautiful man. I have fallen a long way.

MEDITATION ON THE GIVEN

Some beliefs consume you
whole, others piece

by piece. I believe
in nothing as it piles

and piles up, plain
as a pane of glass.

Meditate on the given
and think: isn't this nice?

I confess to sketching
a trajectory on graph

paper and following it,
as close as possible,

in real time. If you want
to get lit, build a fire.

If you want to stroll
through a door,

first approach its threshold.
Enter any room and its great

big nothing gestures
as if to say:

there's an empty chair,
take a seat and we'll begin.

If the chair's not there
all the better.

PABST BLUE RIBBON

After a dry spell it's Pabst,
hissing like a freshly struck
match: 'You can do this good
but no better,' it says.

So I do this good.

Inside the can is a toy piano.
I plunk a few keys
and balloon with dream logic,
airy and untethered music.

The moment lifts its head,

brings word from another season.
But its promises
are strung out, wrung dry,
empty soon enough.

ADVIL CELEBRATES ITS FREEDOM BY FIRING BOTTLE ROCKETS AT THE SKY

When you lose language
something goes blurry
and then you're a county jailor

waiting for your shift to end.
I realized this during my silent phase.
The quiet was milky: a by-product

of grass and growth hormones.
Silence balloons till it pops.
Up next? More silence.

Advil and I want only to singe
the sky's jean jacket
with bottle rockets and call it a day.

I'm haloed by a headache,
like a body's chalky aura.
For weeks, Advil and I loiter in a park,

searching for a cloud that resembles
a plausible end-of-life scenario.
To critics who say my work

is a statement on speech, don't even.
No one asked for this, least of all me.
The difference between a prison

and monastery is where the guards sleep.
Spend too much time on the outside
and your mind goes to seed.

Too much time on the inside and, well,
here we are. The best monks are like poets:
doing very little work.

Read what they've written and you'll find
pages of obscene marginalia. And the middle?
Utterly blank. I use chalk to demonstrate the soul

is an emergent property. Then it rains.
There's no grass in prison, only concrete
someone poured and, God willing, never saw again.

THREE GRACES

for – and after two lines by – Leigh Nash

Regarding the lines in my wife's face:
this one was red, a rose, a rosary.

As an insurance adjuster taps a pen
to express emerging concern,

so do I resolve myself
to hear the good voice saying,

'Faulkner, this isn't about you.'

I made it my hobby to watch
a stranger write my name by hand

until she was no longer strange.
Now what? It's a question

of degree and temperament,
of which I have both. As for a wife's

three graces: to be hem-like
in the way she gathers

the infinitive. To worry a line clean.
And to line up a hundred lies.

The infinitive *settles in with a sigh*:
to pick any lie and true it.

BLOWBACK

Less than perfect. I heard it first
on the CBC. In the background. A whir.
Rattling, like teeth in a bag. A cough?

But constant. Technically in the category
of cultural production. Now I hear it
everywhere. Like that radio song.
With the singer whose voice

is a keystroke. Anyway, it's lurking,
like a pervert. What makes a noise
it shouldn't? A collision of mass.

Stray wire caught in a fan. An object
dragged through space. Audible
topographies. Someone scraping a wall,
digging out. To where?

A click. A bump. There's a name
for it, a definition. A radius.
Local conditions bunch up

and then: *bam*. The brain sits upright.
Thereness that isn't quite there.
When someone enters a room,
loneliness leaves – listen for what blows back in.

SOUND CHECK BEFORE AN ALL-AGES
HARDCORE SHOW IN A YMCA GYMNASIUM

The absence before song: tide when the tide's not in.

The room a graveyard of heavy-metal shirts and undirected attention. As afternoons go, this one is porous. Could swing any which way.

Air runic, silvery with the exhale of a grand human amalgam. Then a screech of feedback leaves the ears candled.

Some kid flicks a switch. The crowd's constituent parts slush and churn. The tide will not be rushed.

The crowd is prepared, purses and backpacks radioactive with malt liquor and Twizzlers. The band has practiced for eons. They steady their weapon-grade thunder and brimstone.

A guy unzips a Fjällräven. In contravention of the gymnasium rental agreement, he proffers a handful of Roman candles. Holds them out like a final, best wish. Lickety split, he's crisp.

Phones emerge and everyone communicates what they need to, and to whom.

The paramedics arrive. The guy, he's a tangle on the floor. His mouth opens, opens again. A wire's cut, a connection fails. No sound comes out.

ADVIL LURKS IN THE LEAVES

Relief's algorithms go sideways.
Pain relinquishes one threshold

for another threshold. Shadows
collect in the eaves. Help, please?

In a year that feels like a shatterwork
of lace, I wash and wash my hands

and face. Advil's abandoned me.
Lurks in the leaves. Drags soot

across every door's frame.
Gnaws away like wind

at weather-stripping.
Advil says three spoons, no,

four spoons of sugar. Wants it
right in its stupid moon face.

Then it'll pull out silver thread
and see what it can do.

SONNET IN WHICH THE TRANSLATOR QUERIES THE AUTHOR

What do you mean by 'submerged'?

Should the reader drown like an untethered feeling or an unattended toddler?

In what way are the saints 'hazy in the middle'?

Do the saints wear their movements like robes?

As for the light: is it bright, slight, or conceptual?

Was the headache a tangle of feet or dense as a Viennese dance hall?

Will you confirm its arc is both inward and 'thick as a waltz'?

The diamond: shape or substance? The gold: filling, plating, or cash?

When the sun 'buries its head like a hatchet,' what type of rest do you mean?

Is the subject crossed like a heart, struck by a mood, or stricken with belief?

Regarding the blood: physical? Metaphysical? Or a special effect?

If Advil 'reconsiders what's given,' on what does it settle?

Where should I locate the centre in this fog of attention?

At what point does pain signal only itself?

RETURN TO SENDER

The coloured wheel that appears
when a user and a slice of Apple's

code disagree is moonlight
swallowed cold. I'm doused in woe.

The wheel practises its scales –
it too has updrafts, collusion

of effort and motive.
For some, death is sudden,

for others a long pause.
My thoughts gather

and plot their return.
If you receive a letter

not yours, you send it back.
You consider the sender.

So I consider the wheel
as it lays down its bouquet.

ADVIL ARRIVES

Above the asphalt morning: a murmur of clouds.
Rail tracks run like two clear thoughts.

The commuter train arrives with a thunk-a-
thunk that paves me over. Like the heart's

fleshy balm – *be better,*
be better – it goes where it goes.

In my skull, nothing's where I left it.
A marble rolls around, an outcome

when the outcome is unknown.
I too want to be parallel.

The sun lays its long hand on my face,
and the breeze finger-puppets

a stand of trees.
Light seesaws which way.

I take two Advil
and round the symptoms up,

count each blistered head
as it passes through the gate.

ON PROPORTION

My face is a darkened door, so what?
I cross a threshold as one might

cross their heart. We are hinged
to our conditions. Caravaggio says

in all paintings the dominant metaphor
is light. When the headache arrives

the weather is an anthem
of silence, teeth clamping a pearl.

Makes you want to sleep
like the dead. According to Seneca,

the greatest obstacle to living
is expectancy. And if I don't expect

to live? Life carries on lightly,
a hum in the background. Things happen

and then happen again. An arch,
a glass tower at dawn, an idle car.

It's embarrassing to worry in detail,
and hard work undoing the self.

My body is a collection of uncoiled
proportions, a thesis that renders

itself obsolete. The five human senses
in their snug dimensions.

Euclid points to a heap of observations
with his are-you-kidding-me face.

I police my headache as it thrashes
in the dead-glass hour. Arrested by the question

of what to do with oneself. Sweep the mind's
chamber clean and then what?

I fold my hands as if they were
a resolution worth keeping.

Caravaggio notes that light stops
where the body starts. How poorly made

we are. How subject to the self's curve
backward into emptiness.

I dearly envy the departed.
But the body, like heaven,

forbids what it doesn't allow.
I unfold my hands as if unlacing

the devil's stitchwork. Gaye's advice
is to sing with one foot in the grave,

according to Abdurraqib. The world
devours its young, anyone can tell

you with a wink. Voices clatter
pots and pans as illness

pitter-patters across the atrium.
Any good contract will stipulate

a proper working order,
which is not what we have here.

Caravaggio says that as mediums go,
you work with what you've got.

Various functions conspire
to entangle into illegibility.

The Old Masters were right
to gaze upon the body's landscape

and say: 'More paint couldn't hurt.'
Like the devil, good health is best known

by its absence. Is it so much to ask,
Woolf wondered, to make the body

a sheet of glass? Take a deep breath
and you'll feel lighter. A buoy,

an empty chair, an unstruck match.
I fold my hands like a flag

claiming jurisdiction
over a modest territory.

Caravaggio says in all paintings
wherever the light strikes

there are two subjects:
the subject, and those

who attend to the subject.
A haze of tension signals

it plans no violence
but will not budge.

Installs an inflatable rat
to watch over the gathering

of human dysfunctions.
A fit of roses, a filament,

a freestone pit. As with grief,
there is no other side.

No proportionate response.
Who doesn't grow weary with being?

I unfold my hands
as if prying my body apart.

Open any door and there I am,
floating along in my orbit

of disrepair with a feverish
conviction to get better

or get out. Like despair,
dying is a useless art.

Good intentions labour in darkness
and so does the devil.

I gather like glitter in dense
little globs. Each sensation flags

an adjacent issue,
that's just what a person is.

Compromised by our vectors,
our situations. An ominous breeze

may blow from any given direction.
Kondo claims a tidy space

leads to transformation
but how do I clean up

a collection of asymmetries
that threaten to sour

the mind? To attend to living
is not necessarily to live.

I fold my hands to indicate
the fit between the life we lead

and the death we get.
Caravaggio, that old nag,

says we should frame light
like a carpenter. Nail down

the details and you'll see
a thing for what it is.

What's the condition of a problem
if you are the problem? I unfold

my hands to show of course
the devil doesn't exist.

God's grace withstanding,
neither will I. Caravaggio says

to picture yourself well
and there you are.

A sparkler, a statement of fact,
an empty preference.

What I love most about my body
is one day it won't be there.

Get the proportions right
and I'll lift myself

into ideation. As for my body,
the future can have it.

NOTES ON THE POEMS

'On Visions,' p. 9: This poem relies on four sources for background information and terminology: *Hallucinations* and *Migraine* by Oliver Sacks; *The Book of Saints*, ed. Dom Basil Watkins, OSB; and catholicsaints.info. The voices of other sources appear verbatim or adapted as follows.

From *Hallucinations* by Oliver Sacks: 'the absence of change may cause a blip in perception'; 'as good and true a sensation' (quoting William James); 'the extraordinary persistence of vision'; 'a fact of shape, orientation, location'; and 'Dogs barking, telephones ringing, a name being called.'

From *In the Land of Pain* by Alphonse Daudet, translated by Julian Barnes: 'smoke against a wall' and 'Like going down two steps at a time.'

From the poem 'Our sermon today concerns the dialectic' from *American Sonnets for My Past and Future Assassin* by Terrance Hayes: 'suffering and ascendance require the same work.'

From the talk 'You and Your Research' by Richard Hamming, which occurred at Bellcore on March 7, 1986: 'go forward under incredible circumstances.'

From *When Things Fall Apart* by Pema Chödrön: 'stay with the shakiness.'

From 'Ecstatic epilepsy: How seizures can be bliss' in *New Scientist*, quoting Dostoevsky: 'A happiness unthinkable in a normal state.'

From the introduction to *The Left Hand of Darkness* by Ursula K. Le Guin: 'anything carried to its logical extreme becomes depressing.'

From the poem 'Black Migraine' from *Green Migraine* by Michael Dickman: 'the saints march through a hole in the sky.'

'Paranoid Android,' p. 24: The phrase 'and say, "Pay your rent and you'll be fine." / Say, "Touch my sister and I'll kill you."' is from my own poem 'Bar Fight,' which originally appeared in *The Fiddlehead* and is otherwise unpublished, with good reason.

'Lichtenberg Cinema,' p. 31: This poem is a mashup of phrases from Ben Lerner's *Lichtenberg Figures* and Lisa Robertson's *Cinema of the Present*.

'Geriatric Millennial Vibes on Nostalgia,' p. 32: The phrase 'pornography of snow' is from the poem 'Two Women on the Potomac Parkway' in *The Mercy Seat* by Norman Dubie.

'Duplicate Worlds,' p. 33: The title comes from the phrase 'The patient enters a duplicate world' in *Illness as Metaphor* by Susan Sontag.

'A Fever Dream May Arrive Despite the Absence of a Fever,' p. 35: The italicized phrases are from *These Possible Lives* by Fleur Jaeggy, translated by Minna Zallman Proctor.

'On Babies,' p. 38: The phrase 'A baby born at twenty-four weeks may weigh just over a pound' is from the story 'The Lesson' from *Get In Trouble* by Kelly Link, and 'plagues begin with rats and fleas' is from *A Thousand Small Sanities: The Moral Adventure of Liberalism* by Adam Gopnik.

'Self-Portrait from Another Room,' p. 40: This poem is indebted to Paul Ford's article 'Just Like Heaven' from *The Morning News*, where I encountered both the phrase 'brain scooped' and the following phrase from the 11th chapter of the *Tao Te Ching*: 'Clay is fashioned into vessels, but it is on their empty hollowness that their use depends.'

'Advil Clumsily Retells Norm Macdonald's Moth Joke from *The Tonight Show with Conan O'Brien*,' p. 49: The original joke is here: afaulkner.ca/moth-joke

'ScroogeMcDuckSwimmingInGoldCoins.gif,' p. 55: 'If love be rough with you, be rough with love' is from *Romeo and Juliet* by William Shakespeare. I got the image of a finger and thumb rubbing to indicate money from the poem 'Your Thought's the Seafoam in the Gyre' in *Safely Home Pacific Western* by Jeff Latosik.

'American Sonnet for my Past and Future Ariel,' p. 61: This poem is a mashup of phrases from Terrance Hayes' *American Sonnets for My Past and Future Assassin* and Sylvia Plath's *Ariel*.

'Meditation on the Given,' p. 62: The title is from the essay 'Reformation' in *The Givenness of Things* by Marilynne Robinson.

'Three Graces,' p. 67: The concept of the 'good voice' is from *Hallucinations* by Oliver Sacks, who also calls it a 'Life voice' and notes that it's an internal voice that guides one out of serious trouble. 'This one was red, a rose, a rosary' and 'settle in with a sigh' are the opening and closing lines, respectively, of the poem 'A Hundred Lies' in *Goodbye, Ukulele* by Leigh Nash.

'On Proportion,' p. 76: The voices of several sources appear verbatim or adapted as follows.

From *On the Shortness of Life* by Seneca: 'the greatest obstacle to living is expectancy.'

From the poem 'Ostinato and Drone' in *Appalachia* by Charles Wright: 'hard work undoing the self.'

From *My Brilliant Friend* by Elena Ferrante: 'How poorly made we are.'

From the essay 'Game of Pearls' in *Figure It Out* by Wayne Koestenbaum: 'curve backwards into emptiness.'

From the poem 'The Ghost of Marvin Gaye Leans Into a Wall Outside The 7-Eleven And Tells You The Story of How He Broke Your Mama's Heart Real Good' in *A Fortune for Your Disaster* by Hanif Abdurraqib: 'Gaye's advice is to sing with one foot in the grave.'

From *On Being Ill* by Virginia Woolf: 'to make the body a sheet of glass.'

From Nick Cave's newsletter *The Red Hand Files* #95: 'as with grief, there is no other side.'

From David Antin's poem 'What it means to be avant-garde': 'the fit between the life we lead and the death we get.'

ACKNOWLEDGEMENTS

Several poems previously appeared in *Canadian Literature*, *Maisonneuve*, *Prairie Fire*, and QWERTY. Many thanks to the editors of these magazines.

I received grants from the Canada Council for the Arts and the Ontario Arts Council that helped me complete this book. I am grateful to the jurors, administrators, and arts workers who run these programs, and to the citizens of Ontario and Canada for funding the arts.

Thanks to Matthew Tierney, who edited this book with a saint's heart and an assassin's eye. Dear reader, where you find soft spots in *Heady Bloom* is where I failed to listen to his advice.

I'm fortunate Alana Wilcox is both my publisher and friend, and I'm endlessly thankful for her deft stewardship of my work. Thanks to Crystal Sikma for the striking cover and interior. Thanks to James Lindsay for connecting *Heady Bloom* with the world outside my head. And thanks to everyone else at Coach House – Tali Voron, Lindsay Yates, and Sasha Tate-Howarth – for the thousand tasks required to produce this book and guide it into readers' hands. Thanks as well to John De Jesus and all the pressfolk for their craft in printing and binding this book.

Leigh Nash carried me through the headache years with tremendous poise, and then I made her spend years reading and re-reading and re-re-reading poems about it all. Leigh, I promise here, in writing, I will never again make you read the words 'a vast pornography of snow.' Thank you for your never-ending support, for making all things possible, and for the boundless pleasure of living my life with yours.

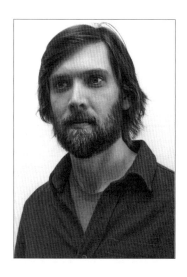

ANDREW FAULKNER is the author of one book of poetry, *Need Machine*, and several chapbooks, one of which was short-listed for the bpNichol Chapbook Award. He has an MFA from the University of Guelph and lives in Picton, Ontario, where he works as the managing editor of Invisible Publishing.

Typeset in Arno and Broadacre.

Printed at the Coach House on bpNichol Lane in Toronto, Ontario, on Zephyr Antique Laid paper, which was manufactured, acid-free, in Saint-Jérôme, Quebec, from second-growth forests. This book was printed with vegetable-based ink on a 1973 Heidelberg KORD offset litho press. Its pages were folded on a Baumfolder, gathered by hand, bound on a Sulby Auto-Minabinda, and trimmed on a Polar single-knife cutter.

Coach House is on the traditional territory of many nations including the Mississaugas of the Credit, the Anishnabeg, the Chippewa, the Haudenosaunee, and the Wendat peoples, and is now home to many diverse First Nations, Inuit, and Métis peoples. We acknowledge that Toronto is covered by Treaty 13 with the Mississaugas of the Credit. We are grateful to live and work on this land.

Edited by Matthew Tierney
Cover art 'hydrangea' by Q-TA
Cover and interior design by Crystal Sikma
Author photo by Tiffany Pope

Coach House Books
80 bpNichol Lane
Toronto ON M5S 3J4
Canada

416 979 2217
800 367 6360

mail@chbooks.com
www.chbooks.com

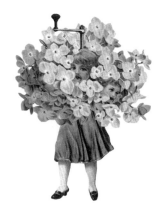